REFLEXOLOGY FOR BEGINNERS

Essential Techniques For Stress Relief, Pain Management, And Holistic Wellness

DR SAWYER DIEGO

DISCLAMER

Nothing in this book should be interpreted as medical advice; it is meant exclusively for educational reasons. Regarding their specific health issues and treatment options, readers are urged to speak with licensed healthcare professionals. The publisher and author disclaim all liability for any errors or omissions in the material provided, as well as for any negative effects that may arise from using or abusing the information. Although every attempt has been taken to guarantee that the material in this book is correct as of the date of publishing, new research may have superseded some of the content because medical knowledge is always changing. It is recommended that readers confirm the most recent medical recommendations and guidelines. The reader of this book undertakes to release the author and publisher from any claims or liabilities resulting from the use of this information, and understands and accepts the inherent risks connected with healthcare decisions.

TABLE OF CONTENTS

ABOUT THE BOOK

"Reflexology for Beginners" is a vital resource for anyone interested in utilizing the holistic advantages of reflexology. It explores the basic principles of reflexology and provides an in-depth look at everything from its historical roots to its contemporary uses. By viewing reflexology as a holistic approach, readers are exposed to its significant impacts on health and well-being. The book also explains the specifics of reflex zones and how they relate to general health, shedding light on how reflexology can be easily incorporated into daily life to enhance well-being.

Throughout, safety precautions and contraindications are carefully outlined to ensure a safe and effective practice environment. The integration of reflexology with complementary therapies like massage and acupuncture underscores its versatility in pain management and stress relief, providing readers with a holistic approach to personal health care. Practicality is a cornerstone of this guide, starting with foundational techniques such as thumb walking and finger walking, essential for anyone beginning their journey into reflexology.

The book's specialized sections address a range of age groups and demographics, stressing safety precautions and customized techniques. Case studies also highlight the effectiveness of reflexology in treating particular conditions, so readers can understand its usefulness in a variety of contexts. Finally, the book delves deeply into the profound effects of reflexology on mental and emotional health, stress reduction, and promoting emotional balance through mindfulness practices.

As they go along, readers learn about reflexology's potential for self-care and personal development, which enables them to create customized wellness plans. Frequently asked questions and answers clarify issues with pain management, hygiene, and how often to schedule sessions. More complex subjects like zone therapy and reflexology in sports and traditional medicine broaden the reader's knowledge, and insights into new developments and trends predict how reflexology will change in the modern healthcare industry.

"Reflexology for Beginners" not only provides readers with useful methods but also cultivates a more profound understanding of the holistic advantages of reflexology. By accepting its tenets and incorporating them into everyday existence, people can improve their quality of life and create the foundation for a revitalized and balanced well-being.

CHAPTER ONE
REFLEXOLOGY OVERVIEW
RECOGNIZING REFLEXOLOGY AS A COMPREHENSIVE APPROACH

Reflexology is a non-invasive, gentle therapy that is often used in conjunction with conventional medical treatments to support overall health and well-being. It is a holistic practice that involves applying pressure to specific points on the feet, hands, and ears to stimulate corresponding organs and systems throughout the body. The ancient healing art of reflexology is based on the idea that these reflex points are interconnected with various parts of the body through energy pathways. By manipulating these points, reflexologists aim to promote balance and facilitate the body's natural healing processes.

Understanding the anatomy of the hands and feet is essential to practicing reflexology effectively. The various areas of the hands and feet correspond to various organs and body systems, including the heart, lungs, digestive system, and more. Reflexologists can help promote physical and mental harmony by relieving tension, enhancing overall relaxation, and improving circulation by applying targeted pressure techniques to these reflex zones.

Reflexology is a form of massage therapy that requires the mastery of specific techniques such as thumb and finger walking, rotating movements, and gentle pressure applications.

The purpose of these techniques is to stimulate nerve endings and encourage the release of endorphins, which in turn promotes relaxation and a sense of well-being. If you are a beginner, practicing on yourself or a willing participant can help you become sensitive to the reflex points and comprehend their therapeutic effects. Sessions last 30 to 60 minutes, which is an adequate amount of time to thoroughly address each reflex area.

REFLEXOLOGY'S HEALTH AND WELLNESS BENEFITS

A holistic therapy, reflexology is believed to support the body's natural healing processes by clearing energy blockages and restoring balance to the corresponding organs and systems. Reflexology offers many benefits for both physical and mental health. By stimulating reflex points on the feet, hands, and ears, this practice can help improve circulation, reduce stress levels, and promote deep relaxation. Many people turn to reflexology to alleviate chronic pain, enhance sleep quality, and boost overall immune function.

Focusing on particular reflex points, reflexologists can help release tension and encourage a state of deep relaxation, which in turn may improve mood and mental clarity. Regular sessions can contribute to better sleep patterns and increased energy levels, as well as improved overall well-being. Reflexology is also known to complement other treatments for various health conditions, offering a holistic approach to wellness. Reduction of stress and anxiety is one of the main benefits of reflexology.

Reflexology is a versatile option for people looking for natural ways to support their health. Whether used as a standalone treatment or in conjunction with conventional medicine, reflexology has shown promising results in improving quality of life and promoting a sense of balance and vitality. For those managing chronic conditions like migraines, digestive disorders, or hormonal imbalances, reflexology can offer relief by addressing underlying issues through gentle pressure and manipulation of reflex points.

EXAMINING THE ORIGINS AND HISTORY OF REFLEXOLOGY

The history of reflexology began thousands of years ago in ancient civilizations like Egypt, China, and India, where it was used as a therapeutic modality. Egyptian tomb paintings from approximately 2500 BC show scenes of physicians treating patients' hands and feet; in China, reflexology was integrated into

Traditional Chinese Medicine (TCM), with an emphasis on stimulating particular points to restore balance and promote health.

The concept of "zone therapy," which proposed that applying pressure to particular zones on the hands and feet could relieve pain and treat various ailments, was developed by American ear, nose, and throat specialist Dr. William Fitzgerald in the early 20th century.

Physiotherapist Eunice Ingham also made significant contributions to the development of reflexology, mapping out the reflex points on the feet and developing the techniques used in modern practice.

Reflexology's historical roots reflect a long-standing belief that the body can heal itself given the right stimulus. By learning about its rich cultural evolution, practitioners can appreciate reflexology not only as a therapeutic modality but also as a testament to the enduring human quest for holistic health practices.

Today, reflexology is recognized as a complementary therapy that can support overall health and well-being.

CRUCIAL EQUIPMENT AND SUPPLIES REQUIRED FOR REFLEXOLOGY PRACTICE

You will need a few basic supplies and tools to ensure comfort and accuracy when practicing reflexology. The first is your hands, which you will use to apply pressure to the reflex points on the hands, feet, or ears.

You should keep your hands clean and your nails clipped to prevent discomfort for you and your client. If you would like, you can use finger cots or gloves for hygienic reasons.

A footstool or leg support can also improve comfort and encourage relaxation during the session. Having cushions or pillows on hand can help adjust positions and provide support where needed. A comfortable reclining chair or massage table is essential for the client's relaxation during the session.

Make sure the chair or table is padded and adjustable to accommodate different body types and preferences.

While some practitioners prefer to work directly on dry skin, it's important to communicate with your client beforehand to ascertain their comfort level and any allergies or sensitivities they may have. Massage oils or lotions can be used to facilitate smooth movements and reduce friction during the reflexology session. Choose hypoallergenic and non-comedogenic products to minimize the risk of skin irritation or allergic reactions.

A supply of disposable wipes or tissues is handy for quick cleanup between clients. With the proper tools and materials prepared, you can create a comfortable and professional environment for your reflexology practice. Clean towels or blankets should be on hand to cover the client and maintain warmth and comfort throughout the session. These can also be used to wipe off excess oils or lotions after the session.

ORGANIZING YOUR WORKSPACE FOR COMFORT AND PRODUCTIVITY

A comfortable chair or massage table with adjustable height settings allows for proper body mechanics and ergonomic positioning during treatments, reducing strain on the practitioner's body and enhancing the client's overall experience. Establishing a quiet, private, distraction-free area where clients can relax and unwind during their session is the first step towards effectively practicing reflexology and ensuring the comfort of both practitioner and client.

A clean and well-organized workspace is essential, with easy access to necessary tools, materials, and hygiene supplies to ensure a hygienic and professional environment. Lighting is important in setting the mood for reflexology sessions. Soft, indirect lighting or natural light helps create a calming atmosphere, promoting relaxation and aiding in the client's ability to unwind.

CHAPTER TWO

REFLEXOLOGY'S BASIS

UNDERSTANDING REFLEXOLOGY

Using pressure on these reflex areas, practitioners hope to induce physiological changes in the corresponding body parts. Reflexology is a holistic therapy based on the theory that various points on the feet (and occasionally hands) correspond to organs, systems, and structures throughout the body. The therapy is predicated on the notion that the body is interconnected and that by adjusting these reflex zones, one can encourages relaxation, enhance circulation, and support general well-being.

Reflexologists work with clients to identify areas of tenderness or imbalance in the reflex zones, which may indicate underlying health issues or areas needing attention.

Reflexology is the practice of applying specific techniques to pressure these reflex points, usually with thumbs, fingers, or specialized tools. The goal is to induce a therapeutic effect in the corresponding area of the body.

The first step in learning reflexology is to become familiar with the anatomy of the hands and feet and how each part corresponds to various organs and systems. Books that describe reflexology maps and techniques or guided instruction can be helpful for beginners. Through practice, people can become more sensitive to touch and learn how to apply pressure in a way that will produce the desired therapeutic effects.

THE THEORY AND FOUNDATIONS OF REFLEXOLOGY

Reflexology is based on several theories, one of which is the idea that the body is made up of energy pathways or zones that run through it. Reflexology theory states that imbalances or blockages in these pathways can cause physical discomfort or illness. By stimulating the reflex points, practitioners seek to remove these imbalances and restore the body's natural healing mechanisms.

Reflexologists believe that by applying pressure to specific points on the hands or feet, they can influence the nervous system and stimulate the body's healing responses. This holistic approach takes into account the interconnectedness of body systems rather than focusing solely on symptoms. Another fundamental idea is that of reflexes and reflex arcs, which are similar to those found in acupuncture and acupressure.

Reflexologists seek to relieve tension, enhance circulation, and assist the body's healing process by promoting relaxation through targeted pressure techniques. This holistic approach addresses both physical and emotional well-being, making reflexology a popular choice for those seeking natural, non-invasive therapeutic methods. The theory underlying reflexology also incorporates principles of relaxation and stress reduction.

THE BODY'S REFLEX ZONES AND HOW REFLEXOLOGY OPERATES

To stimulate the nervous system and encourage balance and healing throughout the body, reflexologists apply pressure to specific reflex zones on the feet and occasionally the hands, which are thought to correspond to organs, glands, and other parts of the body. These reflex zones are mapped out on charts that show the relationship between each area of the foot and its associated body part.

With the toes representing the head and moving downward to include the neck, spine, organs, and extremities, each foot is divided into reflex zones. Reflexologists can address specific health concerns or promote general wellness by applying varying degrees of pressure and using different techniques, such as thumb-walking or circular motions.

Reflexologists can offer targeted therapy and support holistic health goals by refining their techniques through consistent practice and experience.

Reflexologists must have a thorough understanding of the body's reflex zones. To do this, they must become familiar with the reflexology maps and develop sensitivity in their touch to detect subtle changes in the tissues and reflex points.

EXAMINING THE RELATIONSHIP BETWEEN FOOT HEALTH AND GENERAL HEALTH

Reflexologists believe that by working on the feet, they can improve general health and well-being. This method is based on the idea that the feet serve as a mirror of the body's internal organs and systems, reflecting areas of tension, imbalance, or vitality. The feet are important to reflexology because they have reflex points connecting them to various parts of the body.

Reflexologists aim to promote relaxation, relieve pain, and support optimal functioning of organs and systems throughout the body by stimulating specific reflex points on the feet. This further emphasizes the connection between the feet and overall health.

Reflexology can help improve circulation, reduce stress, and enhance the body's natural healing processes.

Reflexology is often used as a complementary therapy alongside conventional medical treatments to support holistic health goals and promote a sense of balance and well-being. Regular sessions can lead to improved energy levels, decreased pain or discomfort, and enhanced overall wellness.

ADVANTAGES OF INCLUDING REFLEXOLOGY IN EVERYDAY ACTIVITIES

Regular practice of reflexology can help lower stress and anxiety levels by promoting relaxation and improving the quality of sleep; it can also help manage pain, especially for chronic illnesses like headaches and back pain. There are many advantages to incorporating reflexology into daily life.

Reflexologists also aim to support detoxification processes and promote the elimination of toxins from the body by stimulating the body's reflex points; this can lead to increased vitality and energy levels. Additionally, reflexology is known to improve circulation, which can support better cardiovascular health and immune function.

Reflexology offers a non-invasive alternative to traditional medical treatments for people seeking natural wellness approaches or managing chronic conditions. It is important to speak with a qualified reflexologist or healthcare provider to create a customized reflexology plan based on each person's needs and goals. Including reflexology in daily life can improve quality of life and maintain general health.

CHAPTER THREE

GETTING REFLEXOLOGY STARTED

FUNDAMENTAL METHODS: FINGER WALKING, THUMB WALKING, AND HOOKING

The basis of any successful reflexology practice is the mastery of fundamental techniques such as thumb walking, finger walking, and hooking. Thumb walking is a technique in which the thumbs are used to walk across the reflex points on the feet, applying gentle pressure in a way that allows for targeted targeting of specific areas corresponding to organs and systems in the body. Finger walking, on the other hand, uses the fingers to navigate smaller, more intricate reflex areas with controlled pressure, making it especially useful for points that may be more difficult to reach with the thumb alone.

Another vital technique is hooking, in which the fingers are hooked around the edge of the foot to enable a deeper, more focused pressure on particular reflex points; novices should concentrate on keeping a steady rhythm and applying constant pressure to guarantee efficacy without creating discomfort. These methods not only enhance the body's natural healing processes and induce relaxation, but they also stimulate circulation and support general well-being.

Consistent practice and refinement of these fundamental techniques will further enhance their therapeutic impact, making reflexology an invaluable tool for promoting holistic health and wellness. Comprehending and applying these fundamental techniques will foster confidence and proficiency in reflexology, enabling practitioners to effectively deliver therapeutic benefits to themselves or their clients.

RECOGNIZING THE FOOT'S PRESSURE POINTS AND REFLEX AREAS

The feet are divided into zones and reflex areas, each of which relates to a specific body part or function.

For example, the tips of the toes correspond to the head and brain, while the heel represents the lower back and intestines. In reflexology, the feet are mapped into specific reflex areas that correspond to various parts of the body, including organs and systems. A thorough understanding of these pressure points and reflex areas is essential for effective practice.

To stimulate the body's natural healing abilities and restore balance, reflexologists target pressure points within these reflex areas during a reflexology session to promote relaxation, improve circulation, and relieve tension. To provide accurate and effective treatments, practitioners should become familiar with the location and sensitivity of each reflex area.

Reflexology offers a holistic approach to maintaining health, emphasizing the interconnectedness of body systems and the therapeutic benefits of touch. Understanding and working with pressure points and reflex areas on the feet requires practice and sensitivity.

As practitioners become more attuned to these areas, they can customize treatments to address specific health concerns or promote overall well-being.

A COMPREHENSIVE GUIDE TO LEADING A REFLEXOLOGY SESSION

A structured approach is necessary to conduct a reflexology session in a way that is both effective and comfortable for the client. Set up a calm and comfortable environment with soft lighting, soothing music, and comfortable seating. Explain the process to the client, highlighting the benefits of reflexology and answering any questions or concerns they may have. Start by feeling for signs of sensitivity or discomfort on the client's feet and adjusting the pressure and techniques accordingly.

To warm up the feet and calm the client, start the session with gentle relaxation techniques like thumb walking or finger circling. Proceed methodically through each reflex area, firming the corresponding points with light pressure; use thumb walking for larger areas and finger walking for more precise points. When deeper pressure is required, incorporate hooking techniques, making sure to check in with the client to determine their comfort level.

Reflexologists can improve their skills and effectiveness in providing therapeutic benefits to clients seeking relaxation, stress relief, and overall health improvement by regularly practicing and refining session techniques. To conclude the session, use gentle strokes and relaxation techniques to promote overall well-being and integration of the treatment; encourage clients to drink plenty of water to help flush out toxins and support the body's healing process.

TYPICAL SYMPTOMS AND SIGNS THAT REFLEXOLOGY CAN TREAT

One of the main advantages of reflexology is stress reduction, as the light pressure applied to reflex points helps release tension and promote relaxation throughout the body. Many clients report improved sleep patterns after reflexology sessions, as the treatment helps calm the mind and body. Reflexology is well-known for its ability to alleviate a variety of common signs and symptoms, promoting overall well-being and relaxation.

By focusing on specific reflex points that correspond to the digestive system, reflexology can also address digestive issues like bloating, constipation, and indigestion. Patients frequently report relief from headaches and migraines after reflexology sessions because the treatment helps to improve circulation and reduce muscle tension in the head and neck areas.

By encouraging the release of endorphins, the body's natural painkillers, reflexology can also help manage pain for conditions like arthritis and chronic pain. It's important to remember that reflexology is a supplement to conventional medical treatments and should not be used in place of professional medical advice or treatment.

By treating these common signs and symptoms, reflexology provides a comprehensive approach to health maintenance and enhances overall well-being for clients seeking natural and non-invasive therapies.

SAFETY MEASURES AND EXCLUSIONS IN THE PRACTICE OF REFLEXOLOGY

Reflexology is generally safe for most people, but to ensure the well-being of their clients, practitioners should be aware of safety precautions and contraindications. For example, clients with open wounds, infections, or foot injuries should avoid reflexology until the wounds have healed. Pregnant women should avoid reflexology during the first trimester as certain pressure points on the feet may stimulate uterine contractions.

To safely customize treatments, practitioners should be transparent with their clients regarding their medical history and any current conditions. Patients with conditions like diabetes, epilepsy, or heart disease should speak with their physician before beginning reflexology to make sure it is a good fit for their specific needs.

Prioritizing client safety and well-being allows reflexologists to provide effective treatments that support overall health and promote relaxation without compromising comfort or exacerbating pre-existing health issues. During a reflexology session, practitioners should use gentle pressure and avoid causing pain or discomfort to the client. Adjust the intensity of techniques based on client feedback and sensitivity levels to ensure a positive and therapeutic experience.

CHAPTER FOUR

METHODS AND TECHNIQUES FOR REFLEXOLOGY

EXTENSIVE ILLUSTRATION OF REFLEXOLOGY METHODS

A holistic approach to wellness, reflexology is a therapeutic practice that involves applying pressure to specific points on the hands, feet, and ears to promote healing and relaxation throughout the body. Each area corresponds to different organs, glands, and body systems, so it's important to set up a comfortable and relaxed environment before beginning. The practitioner should start by using their thumb and fingers to gently press on the reflex points, working systematically from the fingers to the wrist or from the toes to the heel.

Reflexology can be used as a stand-alone therapy or as part of a larger wellness routine. It promotes relaxation and may help with the relief of a variety of ailments.

Firm, steady pressure should be applied to each point, paying particular attention to any areas that feel tender or tense, as these may indicate areas of imbalance in the corresponding body part. To stimulate the reflex points, use circular motions or a back-and-forth movement, adjusting the pressure based on the recipient's comfort level.

USING AROMATHERAPY AND ESSENTIAL OILS IN REFLEXOLOGY

Aromatherapy combined with essential oils can enhance the relaxing effects and therapeutic benefits of reflexology. Essential oils such as lavender, peppermint, or tea tree oil can be applied to the hands of the reflexologist before the session, or a few drops can be placed in a diffuser in the treatment room to create a peaceful atmosphere.

The subtle aroma of the oils can help both the recipient and the giver relax and de-stress as the reflexologist applies pressure to the reflex points.

Aromatherapy can be customized to meet the needs and preferences of each client; different oils have different benefits. For example, lavender is known to be calming and is therefore perfect for relieving stress; peppermint, on the other hand, maybe invigorating and refreshing. Try different blends to see what works best for each reflexology session; adjust the concentration depending on the client's sensitivity and desired effects.

HOW TO USE CHARTS AND MATS FOR REFLEXOLOGY AND OTHER REFLEXOLOGY TOOLS

Reflexology mats are made with textured surfaces that correspond to different reflex points on the feet, providing tactile feedback and enhancing stimulation during sessions. To use a reflexology mat effectively, place it on a flat surface and have the recipient stand or sit comfortably on it, allowing the textured surface to massage the soles of their feet as they shift their weight.

Reflexology tools, such as mats and charts, can help practitioners locate and stimulate reflex points accurately.

During sessions, use reflexology charts—visual aids that show the location of reflex points on the hands, feet, or ears—as a reference guide to identify and target specific areas corresponding to the recipient's health concerns or goals. By combining manual techniques with reflexology tools, practitioners can provide precise and effective treatments catered to individual needs, whether the focus is on relaxation, pain relief, or overall wellness enhancement. Reflexology charts are frequently color-coded to indicate different organs and systems.

TAILORING REFLEXOLOGY SESSIONS TO EACH PERSON'S NEEDS

The process of customizing reflexology sessions entails adjusting the course of treatment to meet the individual goals and preferences of each recipient. To start, a comprehensive consultation is held to gain an understanding of the recipient's medical history, present state of health, and areas of concern. Based on this information, reflex points that correspond to the stomach, intestines, and digestive glands are targeted, and the pressure applied during the session is determined accordingly.

Reflexologists can tailor reflexology sessions to maximize therapeutic outcomes and support overall well-being, fostering a personalized approach to holistic healing. During the session, keep an open line of communication with the recipient to ensure their comfort and provide feedback on areas of tension or tenderness. Some people respond better to gentle pressure, while others may benefit from deeper stimulation.

USING SELF-REFLEXOLOGY TO PROMOTE PERSONAL WELL-BEING

By using the thumb and fingers to apply gentle pressure to reflex points on the hands, feet, or ears—focusing on areas that feel tender or tight—people can experience the benefits of reflexology techniques on themselves, promoting relaxation and supporting overall wellness. To begin, find a comfortable position and create a relaxing environment free of distractions. Work systematically from the toes or fingers towards the heel or wrist, using circular motions to stimulate the reflex points.

Self-reflexology can be incorporated into daily routines as a form of self-care, offering moments of relaxation and stress relief. Experiment with different techniques and pressure levels to find what works best for individual needs and preferences.

By regularly practicing self-reflexology, individuals can support their wellness journey and complement other health practices for a holistic approach to self-care. To enhance relaxation during self-reflexology sessions, engage in deep breathing exercises or incorporate mindfulness exercises.

CHAPTER FIVE

COMBINING REFLEXOLOGY WITH ADDITIONAL THERAPIES

COMPLEMENTARY THERAPIES INCLUDE REFLEXOLOGY, ACUPUNCTURE, AND MASSAGE

Reflexology, acupuncture, and massage are complementary therapies that complement each other to support holistic well-being. Acupuncture, which has its roots in traditional Chinese medicine, uses thin needles inserted into specific body points to stimulate energy flow or qi.

The practices aim to rebalance the body's energy, relieve pain, and address various health conditions. Massage involves manipulating soft tissues to alleviate muscle tension, improve circulation, and induce relaxation. It can range from gentle strokes to deep tissue techniques, catering to different needs like stress relief or injury recovery.

Conversely, reflexology is the practice of applying pressure to reflex points on the hands, feet, and ears that correspond to the body's organs and systems. By stimulating these points, reflexologists seek to facilitate healing, alleviate tension, and enhance overall well-being.

While each therapy has its advantages, their combined benefits increase the efficacy of treating physical ailments and fostering relaxation. Combining acupuncture, massage, and reflexology into a wellness routine can offer comprehensive support for both physical and mental health, meeting the needs and preferences of each individual seeking holistic healing.

THE USE OF REFLEXOLOGY IN PAIN RELIEF AND STRESS MANAGEMENT

Through the application of mild pressure and massage techniques to the hands, feet, or ears, reflexologists can stimulate nerve pathways and encourage the release of endorphins, the body's natural painkillers. This method not only helps with pain relief but also induces a deep state of relaxation, reducing stress levels and promoting overall well-being. Reflexology is a powerful tool in managing pain and alleviating stress because it targets reflex points that correspond to areas of discomfort and tension in the body.

Regular reflexology sessions can be extremely helpful for people with chronic pain conditions like migraines or arthritis because they improve blood circulation and reduce inflammation. Reflexology is a holistic approach that takes into account the interconnectedness of body systems to restore balance and harmony.

People who incorporate reflexology into their wellness routine can benefit from enhanced relaxation and sustained pain management without having to rely solely on medication.

REFLEXOLOGY FOR PARTICULAR ILLNESSES: CONSTIPATION, SLEEPLESSNESS

By stimulating reflex points associated with corresponding organs and systems, reflexology can be specifically beneficial for certain health conditions, such as insomnia and digestive problems. For gastrointestinal disorders, such as irritable bowel syndrome (IBS), reflexologists gently press reflex points related to the digestive tract to improve digestion and ease discomfort. The goal of this therapeutic approach is to restore balance in the digestive system, which may lead to a reduction in symptoms over time with regular sessions.

Similar to this, reflexology sessions specifically designed to address insomnia focus on calming the nervous system and promoting relaxation responses, providing a natural alternative or complement to conventional sleep aids. By stimulating reflex points related to relaxation and sleep regulation, reflexologists help induce a state of deep relaxation conducive to improved sleep quality.

IMPROVING THE BENEFITS OF REFLEXOLOGY WITH DIETARY AND LIFESTYLE ADJUSTMENTS

Adopting a balanced, nutrient-rich diet supports the body's healing processes and enhances the effectiveness of reflexology by providing essential vitamins and minerals. Hydration is also important, as adequate water intake aids in toxin elimination and promotes cellular health, complementing the detoxifying effects of reflexology. These changes in lifestyle and diet are critical to optimizing the benefits of reflexology.

Regular exercise promotes circulation and general vitality, which works in tandem with reflexology's goal of enhancing blood flow and energy flow throughout the body. Stress-reduction methods like yoga or meditation can amplify the relaxation effects of reflexology and support a holistic approach to well-being. Through these lifestyle changes, people can extend the benefits of reflexology beyond sessions and support their journey toward optimal health and vitality.

WORKING TOGETHER WITH HEALTHCARE PROVIDERS: KNOWING WHEN TO GET EXPERT ASSISTANCE

Even though reflexology has many advantages for general health and well-being, it's important to know when to work with healthcare providers on particular medical conditions or issues. Although reflexologists are trained in relaxation, pain management, and general wellness support, they do not diagnose or treat medical conditions. If you have chronic health issues, unusual symptoms, or persistent pain, seeing a healthcare professional guarantees thorough evaluation and appropriate treatment.

When incorporating reflexology into a healthcare plan, communication between the reflexologist and other healthcare providers is necessary to coordinate treatment and optimize results. This cooperative approach guarantees that reflexology effectively supports overall health goals and complements medical treatments; seeking professional assistance is advised when symptoms worsen, medical advice is required, or complementary therapies are being considered in addition to conventional medical care. Together, healthcare providers and reflexologists can offer holistic support that is customized to each patient's needs, promoting well-being and improving quality of life.

CHAPTER SIX

REFLEXOLOGY APPLIED TO PARTICULAR GROUPS

CHILDREN AND INFANTS REFLEXOLOGY: ADVANTAGES AND METHODS

In contrast to adult reflexology, which uses firmer pressure, techniques for children and infants are gentle and soothing, ensuring safety and comfort—important for their developing bodies and sensitive skin—and offer a host of health benefits, including relaxation, improved sleep patterns, and even support for overall well-being. Parents and caregivers can easily learn basic techniques to apply gentle pressure on specific reflex points on the feet or hands, which correspond to various organs and systems in the body. This gentle stimulation can help alleviate common childhood issues like colic, digestive discomfort, and even anxiety.

Recognizing the ease of use and efficacy of these gentle techniques is crucial to comprehending the benefits and techniques of reflexology for children. For instance, applying light pressure with the thumb or finger on reflex points related to the digestive system can help relieve stomachaches or constipation. Reflexology can also be incorporated into daily routines, like bedtime rituals, to improve relaxation and improve the quality of children's sleep. By implementing these techniques, caregivers can offer their children natural, non-invasive support for their health and well-being.

In practice, this means setting up a peaceful space where the child feels safe and at ease. Light tapping or circular motions can be used to apply gentle pressure to the hands or feet, concentrating on areas that match the child's unique needs or symptoms.

By learning these methods and their advantages, caregivers can successfully integrate reflexology into their daily routines, supporting the holistic health and well-being of infants and children.

PREGNANT WOMEN'S REFLEXOLOGY: SAFETY AND COMFORT ISSUES

When reflexology is applied to pregnant women, it can help alleviate common pregnancy-related discomforts like nausea, back pain, and swelling, as well as support the body's natural healing processes. However, it is important to take safety and comfort into consideration.

Light pressure applied to certain reflex points on the hands or feet can help relieve pregnancy-related symptoms and support the body's natural healing processes. However, it is important to avoid certain points that may stimulate uterine contractions, especially during the first trimester.

Reflexology sessions should be gentle and non-invasive, ensuring the mother's comfort and safety at all times. The practice can be integrated into prenatal care routines, offering women a natural and holistic approach to managing pregnancy symptoms.

Reflexology can help make a pregnancy experience positive by promoting relaxation and reducing stress. Expectant mothers should seek the guidance of trained reflexologists who understand the specific points and techniques suitable for each trimester.

Reflexologists can effectively support expectant mothers by adhering to safety guidelines and focusing on their specific needs. The practical application involves using light to moderate pressure on reflex points associated with pregnancy-related discomforts, such as the lower back, digestive system, and hormonal balance. Throughout the session, it is important to pay close attention to the client's feedback and comfort level.

GERIATRIC REFLEXOLOGY: MODIFYING METHODS FOR SENIOR CITIZENS

Reflexologists should modify their approach based on the client's health history and current physical condition, ensuring safety and effectiveness. Geriatric reflexology focuses on gentle stimulation to improve circulation, alleviate pain, and enhance overall well-being. Elderly clients may have sensitive skin and fragile health conditions, requiring a softer touch and shorter sessions.

Session modifications can be made to accommodate mobility issues so that elderly clients are comfortable and relaxed throughout the session. Techniques for geriatric reflexology often involve light pressure on reflex points associated with common aging-related issues such as arthritis, circulation problems, and cognitive decline. By stimulating these points, reflexologists aim to promote relaxation, reduce pain, and support the body's natural healing processes.

Reflexologists should use gentle, slow movements and adjust pressure based on the client's feedback. By focusing on personalized care and tailoring techniques to suit the individual's condition, reflexologists can effectively enhance the quality of life for elderly clients through geriatric reflexology. The practical application involves creating a calm environment and communicating clearly with elderly clients to understand their specific needs and preferences.

REFLEXOLOGY IN PALLIATIVE CARE: FACILITATING COMFORT AT THE END OF LIFE

Reflexology in Palliative Care: Reflexology in Palliative Care recognizes the holistic nature of care, addressing physical, emotional, and spiritual needs during end-of-life stages; the practice focuses on gentle techniques to alleviate pain, reduce anxiety, and promote relaxation; Reflexologists collaborate closely with Palliative Care Teams to incorporate reflexology into comprehensive treatment plans, providing additional comfort and support to patients and their families.

Reflexology for palliative care employs gentle, non-invasive techniques that are customized to the patient's comfort level and preferences. Pain relief, relaxation, and emotional balance reflex points are gently stimulated to promote overall well-being and provide relief. Quiet, calming environments are used during sessions to honor the patient's dignity and foster a sense of peace.

Reflexologists should work closely with the palliative care team, adhering to medical protocols and modifying techniques as necessary. By offering gentle and supportive care through reflexology, practitioners can contribute to the patient's comfort and quality of life during the trying stages of palliative care. Practical application involves compassionate communication and sensitivity to the patient's physical and emotional state.

CASE STUDIES AND TRIUMPHS IN THE FIELD OF SPECIALIZED REFLEXOLOGY

Case studies and success stories from specialized reflexology practices demonstrate the usefulness and advantages of reflexology in a range of health conditions and clientele. By sharing personal accounts of how reflexology techniques have assisted people in managing stress, finding relief from chronic pain, and generally improving their quality of life, reflexologists can bolster the confidence of prospective clients and show the positive effects of reflexology on health and well-being.

Every case study usually includes the client's particular health issues, the reflexology techniques that were employed, and the results that were obtained. Success stories frequently contain testimonies from clients who have seen notable improvements in their general health or symptoms following reflexology treatments; these narratives offer insightful information about the potential advantages of reflexology and inspire others to incorporate it into their holistic healthcare regimen.

Reflexologists can use case studies and success stories to educate the public, advertise their services, and establish credibility in the healthcare industry by documenting and sharing them ethically, respectfully, and with the consent of their clients.

CHAPTER SEVEN

REFLEXOLOGY FOR MENTAL AND EMOTIONAL HEALTH

REFLEXOLOGY'S UNDERSTANDING OF THE MIND-BODY CONNECTION

By applying pressure to these reflex points, practitioners hope to stimulate energy flow and encourage healing within the corresponding areas of the body. Reflexology is based on the theory that certain points on the hands, feet, and ears correspond to organs, systems, and glands throughout the body. This holistic approach emphasizes the interconnectedness of body and mind, viewing health as a harmonious balance between physical and emotional well-being.

This mind-body connection is important to know when practicing reflexology. Reflexologists can help release blocked energy and restore balance by targeting reflex points associated with organs and systems affected by stress or tension.

For example, pressing the reflex point for the adrenal glands, which is linked to stress response, may alleviate tension and promote relaxation throughout the body. This holistic approach not only addresses physical ailments but also fosters mental clarity and emotional stability by promoting a sense of overall well-being.

REFLEXOLOGY METHODS FOR RELAXATION AND STRESS REDUCTION

Reflexology provides a range of techniques designed to effectively reduce stress and induce relaxation. For example, a common technique is to apply light pressure to the solar plexus reflex point, which is on the sole. This helps to reduce stress and anxiety by encouraging deep relaxation and lowering cortisol levels, which are frequently elevated during stressful situations. Another common technique is to massage the diaphragm reflex point, which is located just under the ball of the foot. This can improve respiratory function and release tension in the chest area, which further aids in overall relaxation.

Incorporating these reflexology techniques into a regular self-care routine can help people effectively manage stress levels, enhance relaxation, and improve overall well-being. Another strategy for reducing stress involves stimulating the big toe's pituitary gland reflex point, which may help regulate the body's hormone production and promote a state of calmness and mental clarity.

USING REFLEXOLOGY TO MANAGE DEPRESSION AND ANXIETY

The potential benefits of reflexology in the management of anxiety and depression are becoming more widely acknowledged. Reflexologists target emotional balance and alleviation of symptoms by focusing on reflex points related to emotional health, such as those linked to the brain and nervous system. For example, stimulating the hypothalamus reflex point, which is located at the base of the big toe, may help regulate mood and reduce feelings of anxiety. Applying pressure to the brain reflex point on the toes can promote relaxation and alleviate symptoms of depression by enhancing serotonin and endorphin production.

Reflexology is a gentle yet effective way to promote emotional well-being because it not only targets physical symptoms of emotional distress but also promotes relaxation and stress reduction, which in turn fosters a more balanced emotional state. It can be incorporated into a holistic treatment plan for anxiety and depression to supplement traditional therapies.

ENHANCING MENTAL CLARITY AND EMOTIONAL BALANCE WITH REFLEXOLOGY

Targeting specific reflex points linked to cognitive function and emotional regulation allows reflexology techniques to be customized to improve emotional balance and mental clarity. For instance, applying light pressure to the pineal gland reflex point, which is located on the top of the big toe, may help regulate sleep patterns and promote mental clarity; likewise, stimulating the amygdala reflex point, which is located on the inside of the foot, may aid in processing emotions and lowering emotional reactivity.

Reflexology can be incorporated into mindfulness and meditation practices to help people improve their overall well-being and mind-body connection. When reflexology is combined with mindfulness techniques like focused awareness and deep breathing, it can amplify relaxation responses and support emotional resilience. This integrative approach supports mental clarity by promoting a balanced emotional state and lowering stress levels, which makes it an effective tool for fostering mental clarity and enhancing emotional well-being.

INCLUDING REFLEXOLOGY IN MEDITATION AND MINDFULNESS EXERCISES

Reflexology techniques, such as focusing on reflex points associated with relaxation and mental clarity, can complement meditation by deepening the relaxation response and promoting a sense of inner peace. For instance, applying gentle pressure to the solar plexus reflex point during meditation can enhance relaxation and reduce tension in the abdominal area, facilitating deeper states of mindfulness. By integrating reflexology into mindfulness and meditation practices, one can multiply the benefits of these practices by promoting relaxation, reducing stress, and improving overall well-being.

This integrative approach supports holistic well-being by fostering a deeper connection between body and mind, promoting relaxation, and enhancing overall mental clarity. Reflexology also helps people become more aware of their body's signals and sensations. By focusing on reflex points linked to emotional well-being, such as those associated with the heart and lungs, practitioners can promote emotional balance and enhance mindfulness.

CHAPTER EIGHT

REFLEXOLOGY FOR SELF-CARE AND PERSONAL DEVELOPMENT

THE DAILY SELF-CARE PRACTICE OF REFLEXOLOGY

Finding a quiet, comfortable place to sit back and concentrate on your hands or feet is the first step in practicing reflexology. Start with light massage techniques to warm up the area and increase blood flow. Reflexology offers a comprehensive approach to self-care, using pressure points on the feet, hands, and ears to promote relaxation and overall well-being.

Apply firm but gentle pressure with your thumbs or fingers to specific reflex points that correspond to various organs and systems in the body. For example, you can stimulate the sinus reflex and relieve headaches and congestion by massaging the area just below your toes. Similarly, you can target the heart and lungs by applying pressure to the ball of your foot, which will improve circulation and respiratory function.

Whether you practice reflexology in the morning to energize yourself for the day, during lunch to relieve midday tension, or in the evening to relax and prepare for restful sleep, consistency is key. Once reflexology becomes a regular part of your routine, you'll notice enhanced relaxation, improved mood, and a greater sense of overall well-being. All it takes is 10 to 15 minutes a day.

ESTABLISHING A MORNING, AFTERNOON, AND EVENING REFLEXOLOGY SCHEDULE

To get the most out of reflexology, schedule your sessions according to the different times of day. For example, to stimulate reflex points that support energy and alertness, like the solar plexus and adrenal glands, start your morning sessions with light pressure using your fingertips in circular motions, then gradually increase the intensity to awaken your senses and get ready for the day.

When the afternoon wears on, work on reflex points related to relaxation and stress release. Concentrate on the diaphragm and adrenal glands to release tension and improve mental clarity. Use deep breathing exercises to enhance the relaxing effects of reflexology and help you feel more focused and productive for the rest of the day.

After dinner, proceed to a calming reflexology session designed to help you unwind and get ready for bed. Focus on reflex points associated with the pituitary and pineal glands to help you fall asleep and feel deeply relaxed. Use slow, rhythmic strokes with light pressure to help release endorphins and serotonin, which will help you get a good night's sleep and guarantee that you wake up feeling renewed and rested.

METHODS OF REFLEXOLOGY FOR INCREASING VITALITY AND ENERGY

Practices that focus on reflex points that correspond to the adrenal glands and thyroid gland, which are located on the tops of the feet and the base of the big toe, respectively, can be especially helpful for beginners who want to improve their general well-being. Firmly press these reflex points with your thumbs in a kneading motion to stimulate the adrenal glands and raise your energy levels.

Reflexology can be incorporated into your daily routine as needed to combat fatigue and improve vitality.

You may also choose to incorporate reflexology sessions during work breaks or before physical activity to maximize performance and stamina.

Reflexology can help you achieve a balanced flow of energy and improve general vitality by focusing on specific reflex points linked to energy pathways in the body, such as the sacral reflex and solar plexus.

As you gain more experience with energy-boosting reflexology techniques, try varying the pressure and massage strokes to see what feels good for you. To get the most out of reflexology for sustained energy and vitality throughout the day, stay hydrated and takes breaks as needed.

HOW REFLEXOLOGY CAN ENHANCE LIFE QUALITY IN GENERAL

By stimulating reflex points that correspond to different organs and systems in the body, reflexology provides a natural and non-invasive way to improve overall quality of life. Whether you're a beginner or an experienced practitioner, reflexology can help reduce stress, promote relaxation, and improve physical and mental well-being.

You can help create a sense of balance and harmony within the body by applying pressure to specific reflex points on the hands, feet, or ears.

By targeting reflex points associated with the digestive system, such as the stomach and intestines, reflexology can support healthy digestion and ease symptoms of gastrointestinal discomfort. Stimulating reflex points linked to the nervous system can help reduce anxiety, improve sleep quality, and enhance mood. Regular practice of reflexology can also contribute to better circulation, reduced tension in muscles and joints, and improved immune function.

Whether you practice reflexology at home or under the supervision of a certified reflexologist, incorporating reflexology into your routine can help you reap the cumulative benefits over time and take charge of your health and well-being.

Reflexology can improve your quality of life overall by fostering a stronger connection between your mind and body, which can lead to a greater sense of vitality and inner balance.

CREATING YOUR OWN CUSTOMIZED REFLEXOLOGY PROGRAM FOR LONG-TERM GAINS

Creating a customized reflexology plan will maximize its long-term benefits and support your overall health and wellness objectives. Begin by identifying specific areas that you would like to see improved, such as energy levels, stress management, or general relaxation. Speak with a qualified reflexologist or consult resources to find out which reflex points correspond to these areas, then create a targeted approach to address them.

Make a plan that incorporates reflexology sessions into your weekly schedule; choose morning or evening times depending on your preferences and lifestyle; emphasize consistency and slow advancement; begin with shorter sessions and extend them over time as you gain comfort with the techniques; maintain a record or journal to monitor your progress and record any alterations or enhancements in your mental or physical health.

To enhance the benefits of reflexology and deepen your practice, you can experiment with different techniques or explore advanced methods. By being proactive in your reflexology practice, you can create a routine that will support your long-term health and well-being and enable you to achieve optimal balance and vitality in your daily life.

CHAPTER NINE
FREQUENT QUESTIONS AND CONCERNS IN REFLEXOLOGY
HANDLING PAIN AND UNEASE DURING SESSIONS OF REFLEXOLOGY

When receiving reflexology, you may feel anything from mild discomfort to occasional pain, particularly in areas that correspond to clogged or unbalanced organs. This discomfort usually indicates areas where an energy blockage or imbalance needs to be addressed, and reflexologists use techniques like slow, gentle pressure application and light massage to address this.

Clients and practitioners need to communicate so that your reflexologist can adjust pressure and technique accordingly. It should be noted that although reflexology can occasionally be slightly uncomfortable, it should never be extremely painful. If pain continues or gets worse during a session, you should notify your practitioner.

HOW FREQUENTLY SHOULD REFLEXOLOGY BE PRACTICED?

The frequency of reflexology sessions varies depending on the needs and goals of each client; weekly sessions are generally advised for general relaxation and well-being; more frequent sessions, perhaps two or three times a week at first, and then progressively fewer as symptoms improve; consistency is essential in reflexology practice; regular sessions support overall health and balance; you should pay attention to your body; if you feel any discomfort or fatigue after a session, you may need to adjust the frequency or duration of sessions. Speaking with a qualified reflexologist can help you create a customized schedule that fits your lifestyle and health goals.

TECHNIQUES FOR MODIFYING FOR VARIOUS FOOT TYPES AND SENSITIVITIES

Reflexologists are trained to assess foot conditions and tailor their approach accordingly.

They may use tools like charts and diagrams to accurately identify reflex points and apply techniques that suit individual foot structures. Adapting techniques ensures that reflexology remains a beneficial and enjoyable experience for clients of all foot types and sensitivities. For those with thicker skin or less sensitivity, slightly firmer pressure may be needed to effectively stimulate reflex points.

MAINTAINING SANITATION AND HYGIENE IN THE PRACTICE OF REFLEXOLOGY

Reflexologists must adhere to stringent hygiene and sanitation protocols to prevent the spread of infections and guarantee client safety. They should wash their hands thoroughly before and after each session, use fresh towels or disposable covers on massage chairs or tables, and disinfect equipment and surfaces between clients to maintain a sterile environment. Clients can also help with hygiene by making sure their feet are clean before sessions and informing their reflexologists of any skin conditions or infections.

By putting hygiene and sanitation first, reflexologists create a safe and hygienic environment that promotes their clients' health and well-being.

OVERCOMING SKEPTICISM: PROOF AND STUDIES IN FAVOR OF REFLEXOLOGY

Since reflexology works on the basis that reflex points on the feet correspond to specific organs and systems in the body, reflexologists aim to stimulate circulation and promote natural healing processes. Knowing the evidence and research behind reflexology can help alleviate skepticism and encourage people to practice reflexology. Reflexology has gained recognition for its therapeutic benefits, supported by research indicating its effectiveness in promoting relaxation, reducing pain, and improving overall well-being. Studies have shown that reflexology can help alleviate symptoms of conditions such as migraines, anxiety, and chronic pain.

CHAPTER TEN

EXAMINING TOPICS IN ADVANCED REFLEXOLOGY

ADVANCED METHODS: ZONE THERAPY AND CROSS REFLEXOLOGY

Advanced reflexology methods such as cross-reflexology and zone therapy entail a deeper comprehension of the reflex zones on the hands and feet. Cross-reflexology incorporates the ideas of zone therapy by emphasizing reflex points that intersect various body zones. This method postulates that certain points on the hands and feet correspond not only to particular organs but also to parts of the body that may have similar neural pathways or functional relationships.

Learning cross-reflexology requires a detailed understanding of the reflex zones and diligent practice to locate and treat these cross points accurately. Practitioners of cross-reflexology use a systematic approach to identify these cross points and apply targeted pressure or massage techniques to stimulate them. By doing so, they aim to enhance the overall therapeutic effects of reflexology, promoting relaxation, and stress relief, and possibly aiding in the management of specific health conditions.

The integration of cross-reflexology with zone therapy improves the practitioner's capacity to address complex health issues and provide targeted relief to their clients. Zone therapy, on the other hand, focuses on specific longitudinal zones running from the feet to the head, each associated with specific organs and body systems. Reflexologists believe they can stimulate energy flow and promote healing in corresponding parts of the body by applying pressure to these zones.

REFLEXOLOGY FOR ENHANCING ATHLETIC PERFORMANCE AND HEALING INJURIES

Applying reflexology techniques to athletes' physical well-being and injury recovery is known as reflexology for sports performance and injury recovery. This method, which differs from general relaxation reflexology, focuses on particular reflex points that correspond to the muscles, joints, and organs that are essential to athletic performance. By stimulating these points, reflexologists hope to increase circulation, lessen muscle tension, and hasten the healing process following intense physical activity or injury.

Reflexologists trained in sports reflexology understand the biomechanics of movement and the impact of sports-related stress on the body. They customize their treatments to support the athlete's training regimen, focusing on areas such as the feet (which bear the brunt of physical exertion), hands, and occasionally even the ears, where reflex points for different parts of the body are believed to be mirrored. Athletes frequently seek reflexology sessions to enhance their overall performance by addressing specific areas of tension or discomfort related to their sport.

Reflexology helps athletes maintain optimal physical conditions and supports their overall well-being during intense training periods and competitive seasons. It can be incorporated into sports recovery programs in addition to other therapeutic modalities like physical therapy and massage.

MERIDIANS IN TRADITIONAL CHINESE MEDICINE (TCM) AND REFLEXOLOGY

The philosophy of energy flow and balance within the body is shared by both reflexology and Traditional Chinese Medicine (TCM) meridians. TCM views meridians as energy pathways that allow Qi (life force energy) to flow, nourishing and regulating the body's organs and systems. TCM-trained reflexologists apply this knowledge to reflexology by identifying reflex points that correspond to particular meridians and their associated organs in addition to physical structures.

Reflexology practitioners trained in TCM meridians may incorporate additional techniques such as acupressure or meridian tracing during sessions to enhance the therapeutic effects of their treatments. By stimulating these reflex points, reflexologists seek to harmonize the flow of Qi, resolve blockages, and restore balance within the body. This holistic approach takes into account the interconnectedness of body systems and emphasizes preventive care as well as treatment of existing health conditions.

Reflexologists need to be well-versed in TCM meridians to locate reflex points that correspond to particular meridians and use the right techniques to promote overall health and wellness. This requires a thorough understanding of both reflexology maps and TCM principles.

AYURVEDA AND REFLEXOLOGY: COMBINING EASTERN HEALING METHODS

Reflexology and Ayurveda both take a holistic approach to health and well-being, emphasizing the body's natural healing processes and balancing energy fields.

Ayurveda is an ancient Indian medical system that divides people into three constitutional types (Vata, Pitta, and Kapha), each of which is associated with unique physical, emotional, and mental characteristics. Reflexologists who have studied Ayurveda can tailor treatments to each patient's dosha and current health needs.

The goal of Ayurvedic reflexology is to balance the doshas, reduce imbalance symptoms, and enhance general health and vitality by stimulating reflex points that correspond to the organs and systems associated with each dosha. This customized approach takes into account not only physical symptoms but also the individual's constitution and lifestyle factors that may have an impact on their health.

By combining these Eastern healing practices, reflexologists can provide holistic care that addresses the underlying causes of imbalance and supports the body's innate ability to heal itself. Reflexologists who integrate Ayurvedic principles into their work must understand the dosha system and its implications for health and wellness. They may suggest dietary changes, lifestyle adjustments, or herbal remedies in addition to reflexology treatments to support the client's journey toward optimal health.

PROFESSIONAL DEVELOPMENT AND ONGOING EDUCATION IN REFLEXOLOGY

Reflexology is a dynamic field where new techniques, research findings, and ethical considerations constantly evolve. Continuing education programs offer opportunities for reflexologists to deepen their knowledge, expand their repertoire of techniques, and explore specialized areas such as prenatal reflexology, reflexology for children, or advanced therapeutic applications.

Professional development and continuing education are essential for reflexologists seeking to enhance their skills, stay updated with industry trends, and maintain high standards of practice.

In addition to continuing education in anatomy, physiology, pathology, and client care, reflexologists can further their professional development by participating in workshops, seminars, and conferences where they can pick the brains of seasoned practitioners and authorities in related fields. These events not only help reflexologists advance their clinical skills but also promote networking within the reflexology community and expose them to a variety of viewpoints on holistic health care.

Continuous education also assists reflexologists in keeping up with certification and licensure requirements, guaranteeing that they adhere to legal requirements and professional standards in their work. Reflexologists who stay up to date on emerging research and best practices are better able to provide their clients with efficient, evidence-based care and further the field of reflexology as a respected complementary therapy.

CHAPTER ELEVEN

UPCOMING DEVELOPMENTS AND TRENDS IN REFLEXOLOGY

NEW DEVELOPMENTS IN REFLEXOLOGY EQUIPMENT AND TOOLS

Over the past few years, there have been notable technological advancements in the field of reflexology to improve both the therapeutic outcome and the client experience. One such development is the creation of sophisticated reflexology tools and equipment. While traditional reflexology tools such as wooden sticks and massage balls have been replaced by cutting-edge devices like electric foot massagers and reflexology sandals, these new tools are specifically made to target specific reflex points, giving clients more effective stimulation and relaxation.

As technology advances, we can anticipate more integration of AI and machine learning into reflexology devices, potentially offering personalized treatment plans tailored to individual health profiles. In addition, there has been an increase in the use of digital technologies to support reflexologists in their practice. Mobile apps and software programs now offer reflexology mapping, allowing practitioners to quickly locate and treat reflex points based on client-specific needs. These technologies not only streamline the reflexology process but also enhance communication between practitioners and their clients by providing detailed reports and progress tracking.

The incorporation of new technologies into reflexology tools and equipment is a major step toward improving therapeutic results and client satisfaction.

These developments not only raise the bar for more individualized and technologically advanced holistic healthcare practices, but they also increase the accuracy and efficacy of reflexology treatments.

RESEARCH ON REFLEXOLOGY AND ITS EFFECT ON CONTEMPORARY HEALTHCARE

Recent studies have examined the physiological mechanisms underlying reflexology and confirmed its ability to induce relaxation, reduce pain, and improve circulation. This scientific validation has bolstered reflexology's credibility within the healthcare community and led to its inclusion in integrative medicine approaches. Research on reflexology has gained momentum, driving its integration into modern healthcare practices and validating its therapeutic benefits.

Beyond these traditional applications, research on reflexology has also looked into how it might be used to manage chronic conditions like diabetes, hypertension, and chronic pain syndromes. The results of these studies have been encouraging, suggesting that reflexology can be used in conjunction with traditional treatments to help patients live better lives by reducing symptoms and improving their overall quality of life. As research methods continue to advance, such as randomized controlled trials and neuroimaging studies, we should anticipate learning more about the neurobiological underpinnings of reflexology's therapeutic effects.

Finally, reflexology research bridges the gap between traditional practices and modern medical standards, positioning reflexology to play a critical role in integrative health approaches of the future. In summary, research on reflexology continues to influence modern healthcare by offering evidence-based support for its therapeutic benefits and expanding its application in managing various health conditions.

TRENDS IN CERTIFICATION AND EDUCATION FOR REFLEXOLOGY WORLDWIDE

A growing number of accredited reflexology training programs are available worldwide, providing structured curricula covering anatomy, physiology, reflexology techniques, and practical hands-on training. The goal of these programs is to ensure competency among reflexologists and standardize education, thereby preparing them for professional practice and certification. Notable developments have occurred in the global landscape of reflexology education and certification, reflecting growing interest and professionalization within the field.

Furthermore, an increasing number of reflexologists are becoming certified online, which has led to a rise in the number of certified reflexologists and the global recognition and acceptance of reflexology as a valid healthcare practice. Online platforms allow for schedule flexibility and high-quality education from recognized institutions without geographical limitations, which has made education more accessible to those who aspire to become reflexologists worldwide.

In summary, the development of reflexology education and certification is a response to the increasing demand for certified reflexologists and standardized training programs across the globe.

The field is expanding its reach and professionalizing its practitioners worldwide by adopting online learning platforms and upholding strict accreditation standards.

INTEGRATIVE HEALTH AND WELLNESS CENTERS' USE OF REFLEXOLOGY

Reflexology complements other wellness modalities like massage therapy, acupuncture, and yoga by addressing both physical and emotional aspects of health. Integrative health and wellness centers are adding more and more reflexology to their service offerings as they recognize its therapeutic value and holistic benefits. These centers offer a supportive environment for clients seeking comprehensive healthcare solutions, encouraging synergy among various modalities to enhance overall well-being.

Reflexologists aim to restore balance within the body's systems by stimulating reflex points on the hands and feet, which promote relaxation, reduce stress, and supports immune function.

This holistic approach resonates with clients seeking natural and non-invasive therapies that support their wellness goals. Furthermore, reflexology plays a role in integrative healthcare that goes beyond symptom management to preventive care and health maintenance.

To sum up, the incorporation of reflexology into integrative health and wellness centers highlights its role as an important part of holistic healthcare practices. These centers represent the future of patient-centered care because they provide integrated treatment plans and encourage collaboration among various healthcare professionals.

THE FUTURE OF HOLISTIC HEALTHCARE: THE INFLUENCE OF REFLEXOLOGY

As part of a holistic approach to health, reflexology addresses the interconnectedness of mind, body, and spirit by stimulating reflex points that correspond to various organs and systems in the body. This therapeutic intervention not only promotes relaxation and stress reduction but also supports the body's natural healing processes. Reflexology is becoming more and more recognized as a crucial element in shaping the future of holistic healthcare, emphasizing prevention, wellness, and patient empowerment.

Reflexology is also a good fit for a variety of people, including those who are seeking preventive care or managing chronic conditions, because it is non-invasive and can induce deep relaxation. Integrative healthcare models support reflexology in addition to conventional medicine, emphasizing its role in promoting wellness-oriented lifestyles and improving overall quality of life.

Finally, reflexology's incorporation into holistic healthcare practices highlights how it can help shift the paradigm toward patient-centered care and preventive health strategies.